The Magic of Turmeric

For Health and Beauty

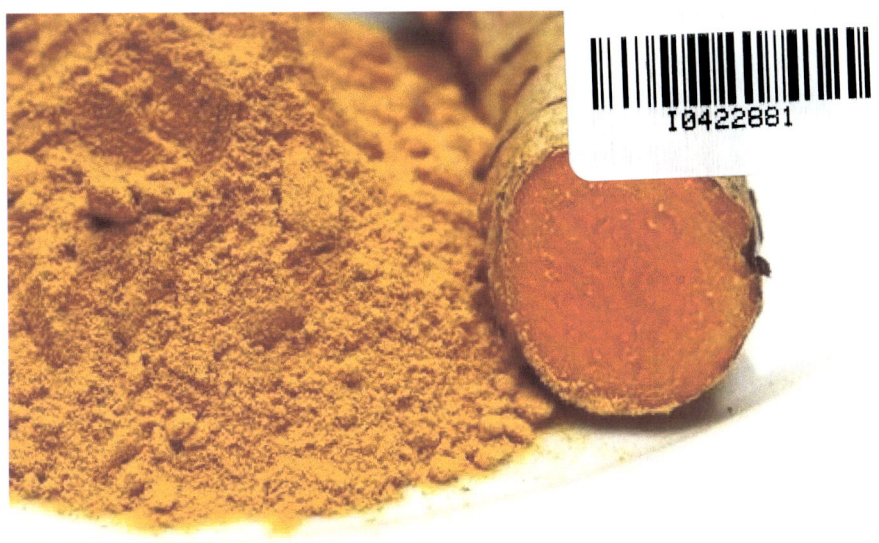

Dueep Jyot Singh

Natural Remedy Series

Mendon Cottage Books

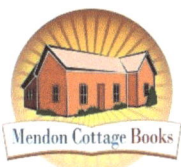

JD-Biz Publishing

Disclaimer

The information is this book is provided for informational purposes only. It is not intended to be used and medical advice or a substitute for proper medical treatment by a qualified health care provider. The information is believed to be accurate as presented based on research by the author.

The contents have not been evaluated by the U.S. Food and Drug Administration or any other Government or Health Organization and the contents in this book are not to be used to treat cure or prevent disease or mental illness.

The author or publisher is not responsible for the use or safety of any diet, procedure or treatment mentioned in this book. The author or publisher is not responsible for errors or omissions that may exist.

Warning

The Book is for informational purposes only and before taking on any diet, treatment or medical procedure it is recommended to consult with your primary care provider.

Our books are available at

1. Amazon.com

2. Barnes and Noble

3. Itunes

4. Kobo

5. Smashwords

6. Google Play Books

Table of Contents

Introduction

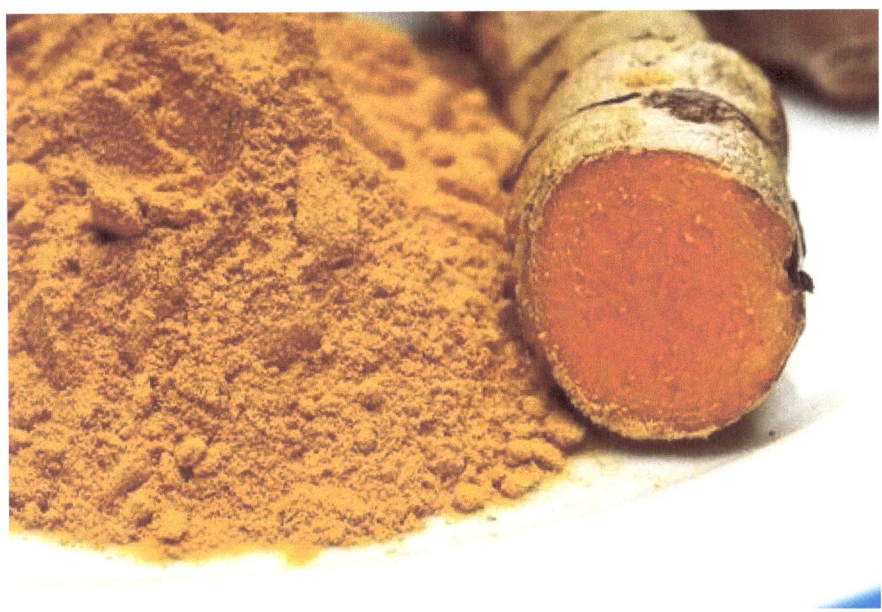

There is an ancient and amusing saying, very prevalent in the East," Mr. Rat found a rhizome of turmeric; he immediately opened up a grocers/herbalist shop!" This may be used to talk about a dreaming, ambitious person, who is trying to extend his wings beyond his capacities, but on the other hand, it talks all about the power of turmeric.

As a grocer, Mr. Rat could not only sell turmeric as a condiment and as a spice, for cooking purposes, but he also had easy access to the cure-all for all ailments – turmeric!

Scientific research in the West, has found out that turmeric, has antibiotic and germicidal qualities, but that was already known in the ancient alternative medicine of the Orient and of the East. It had to be a necessary part of the medical arsenal of every wise woman out there, in ancient times, because if she did not have easy access to the medicine man or to a physician, she just had to resort to plain old turmeric.

So her family's cough and cold prevalent chest infections, cuts, wounds, and even skin problems in her teenage kids, with those pimples and skin blemishes could be cured by turmeric.

The idea that turmeric is used just as a spice, giving flavor and a golden color to cuisine, is slowly and steadily disappearing from the Western mind. Instead, they are getting to know more about its curative properties, thanks to research telling them about Curcumin – a natural product present in turmeric, which keeps you safe, healthy, and also prevents cancer.

Chinese, Greek, Egyptian, Indian, and Oriental medicine knew all about the value of this rhizome since ancient times. This plant belongs to the same family as the equally important curative Herb – ginger.

The herb that you are going to get in the market, is going to be a golden yellow powder, made up of grinding dry rhizomes in a heavy-duty grinder.

I remember one of the persuasive salesman, trying to persuade my father to buy some of his hundred percent pure, freshly ground in his own mill turmeric powder, packaged in his own shop. My father looked at him and told him, "last time I bought some of this hundred percent pure, freshly packaged powder from the market, I put a teaspoon full of it in the water, and I have got enough of saffron dye mixed in it to dye a turban!" That shut the sales man up, because that is when guilty conscience works.

Yes it is true; the powder that you are going to get in the market today is possibly definitely not pure, that is why it is necessary for you to use a grinder to grind the rhizomes.

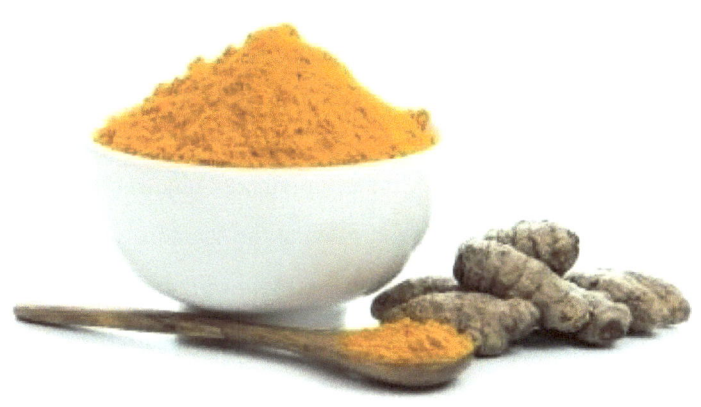

This book is going to tell you all about the magic of turmeric, and you are going to be surprised to know that you knew so less about this amazing herb/spice. Not only is it being used extensively to cure and prevent life-threatening diseases, but it can help save you a lot of headaches and possible financial expenditure, related to your health in the future.

There Is Something about Turmeric

Turmeric is supposed to be a native of Indonesia and southern India. More than 5000 years ago, this herb was being discussed extensively in ancient Siddha medicine, the traditional alternative medicine of South India.

That reminds me of a very interesting mythological figure of Kerala – Tacholi Othenan. He is considered to be a legendary warrior, who even surpassed his master in sword fighting. Well, one fine day he and his brother and the rest of his friends were just strolling about in the village, when they saw a group of lovely ladies just passing by.

Amidst them was one who was extremely plain and unattractive. Othenan could not resist a snide remark of "golly what the scarecrow. She should hire herself out to the Moplah (Mussalman trader of the city) to guard his drying copra." And away they went, very well pleased with themselves, but the girls did not mind going to the mother of plain Jane and telling her what remarks her daughter had to hear.

Mom was a traditional Wise woman. She immediately began to use Natural remedies with herbs and spices to start the beautification process of her daughter.

Within 6 months her daughter was an acknowledged Beauty of the city, in a city of known beauties.

(For all those people who give a cynical grin on reading this , friends, it is true. This ancient aromatherapy, naturopathy and other local remedies have been used by men and women of that area for millenniums to keep them young healthy and beautiful. The herbs which were used to make her skin soft, healthy and beautiful was of course turmeric with milk or cream. Her lanky and lusterless hair would grow silky and long, with powdered Indian gooseberry, Shikakai and soap nut. She would use homemade Kohl to make her eyes look mysterious and lovely. Her skin would be massaged with coconut oil until it was soft and silky. And so on. All this was, of course proud and indignant mama's effort, who finally woke up to the fact that her daughter was not attractive in the eyes of eligible suitors .)

Well, it so happened that about eight months later, Othenan happened to see her walking back with her friends, and definitely not recognizing her, asked his brother to find out who that beauty was. Because of course he intended to make her the queen of his home, heart and Hearth.

In answer, that spirited lady said, "tell your friend that I am just coming back from the Moplah's where I was busy guarding his drying copra. And I want nothing to do with him."

Of course, it is a happily ever after because after a bit of apologizing and groveling, she accepted his hand in marriage. In Kerala, it is the girl who says yes. Anyway, the next morning, the elder brother could not resist shouting triumphantly at the door of mother dear, "Your daughter has accepted the hand of my brother in marriage. Hurray, hurray." And then he had to run for his life throughout the city because mom picked up the nearest chopper and followed him, intent on mayhem. Nevertheless, her daughter became the very well cherished wife of that legendary warrior, Tacholi Othenan.

So if one considers oneself plain and does not intend to improve one's looks or personality, that is his or her outlook. On the other hand, if you are willing to work on it with natural remedies, you can start with turmeric!

How to Grow Turmeric

Curcuma Longa best flourishes in tropical regions, so if you are living in an area where there is a harsh winter and hoarfrost, you will have to plant your turmeric indoors.

That is because this is a perennial plant, and it is going to be dormant in the winter. But with the coming of spring, you're going to have fresh new turmeric shoots springing up and fresh new plants growing.

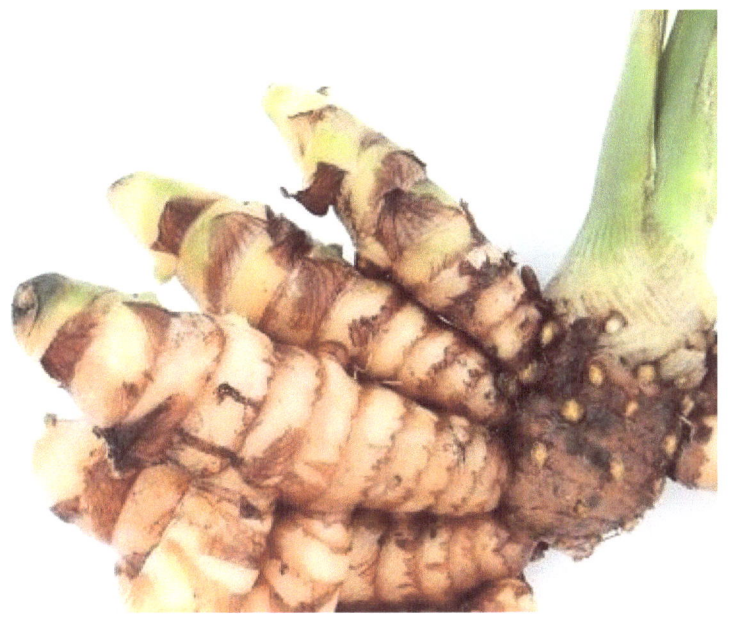

It is rather difficult to grow turmeric from seeds, so you can leave that process to the horticulturists. Instead, look for rhizomes which are fresh, and definitely not infected with fungus. The best rhizomes, like ginger rhizomes ready for planting are going to have one or two small shoots coming out of them.

Cut these portions, very carefully and make your soil ready for turmeric.

Best Soil for Turmeric

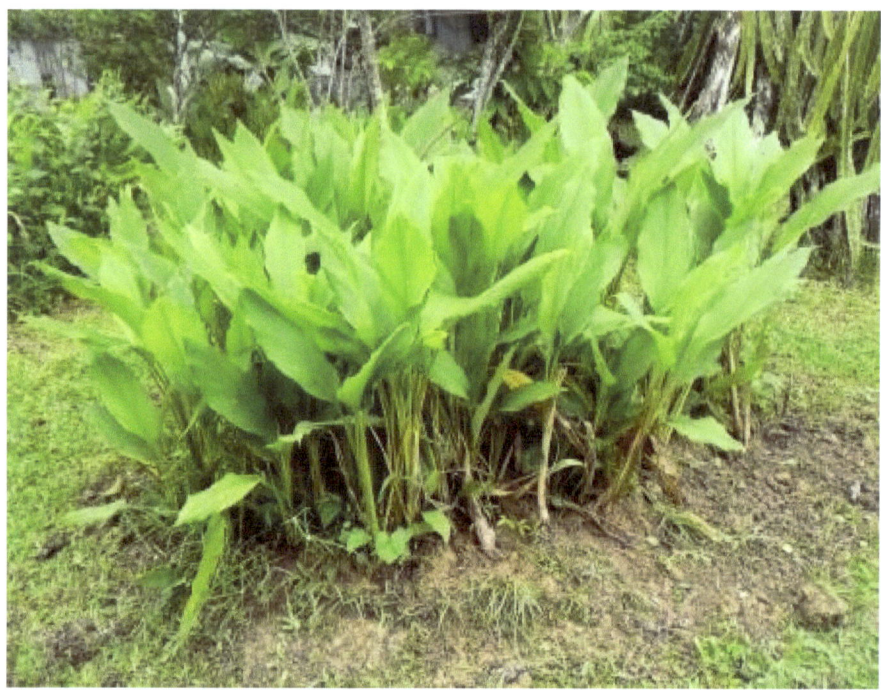

Any sort of soil can do for turmeric as long as it is well drained, and there is plenty of water, and sun around. Apart from tropical zones, turmeric is also going to do very well in the USDA, sunny zones, especially 7 to 10 B zones.

You are going to plant them in either direct sun, when the sun is not so harsh or in indirect sun, when the afternoon sun is bold and brassy, when it reaches its zenith.

If you are living in a tropical zone, you can plant this anytime. But the preferred planting time is spring, after the frost is over. You may also plant the fresh roots in the soil, directly. In fact, villagers in the East keep some dried rhizomes from their previous year's harvest, to plant in the next planting season.

How to Harvest Turmeric

It is going to take up to 40 days to 60 days for the shoots to appear, so be patient. 10 months after the shoots have appeared, you can harvest your turmeric crop. That is when the stems and the leaves start drying up after flowering.

You are going to dig up the full plant along with the root. Calculate the time taken – 60 days for shoot appearance and 10 months for crop to get ready, so that you can plant this at a time when you can harvest it in summer.

Turmeric is traditionally dried by boiling the roots for 45 minutes. Then it is put into the sun to dry and become a dry rhizome. You can also use raw and fresh turmeric in its grated form.

Every plant is going to give you about half a kilo to 750 g of turmeric.

Turmeric Essential Oil

Just like ginger, turmeric also uses an essential oil which is very useful in making ointments for sprains, skin problems, fungal infections, muscular pains and joint pains, as well as curing athletes foot.

One note please – if you are suffering from diabetes and are taking drugs, which lower your blood sugar, Never eat turmeric. Both are mutually incompatible.

Storing Your Turmeric

If you have already got a harvest of turmeric rhizomes, you need to make sure that they are stored in a place, which is completely dry and without moisture. This storage area is best in sand, where your turmeric rhizomes will not have to bother about infection, fungus and moisture. That is why other rhizomes like ginger are also preserved in sand for a long while.

When you go collecting turmeric for preservation at home, make sure that the rhizomes that your green grocers are fresh. They should give a soft odor which is a mixture of oranges as well as ginger.

You can always chop a little bit of these rhizomes, and use it instead of turmeric powder, because you are waiting for the rhizomes to dry out in the sun, before you grind them into real honest-to-goodness home ground turmeric.

Sun-dried turmeric is best kept in airtight containers in a dark and shady place. You may want to air them occasionally in the sun, so that any possibility of moisture and fungus dies at the very onset itself.

How to Grind Turmeric

Traditionally, the duty of grinding turmeric, was given to someone who you wanted to punish. He was given lots of dry rhizomes, and told to roll up his sleeves. After that, he would be given a pestle and mortar, and put to work to make the course powder or a fine powder, depending on the finicky nature of the cook. Well, we are lucky that we are not living in ancient times, and have access to heavy-duty grinders.

So you are going to take the rhizome, chop it into manageable pieces, and roast it gently over a dry griddle. After that, you are going to take this roasted turmeric, and put it in your heavy-duty grinder. Allow for either coarse grinding or for fine grinding.

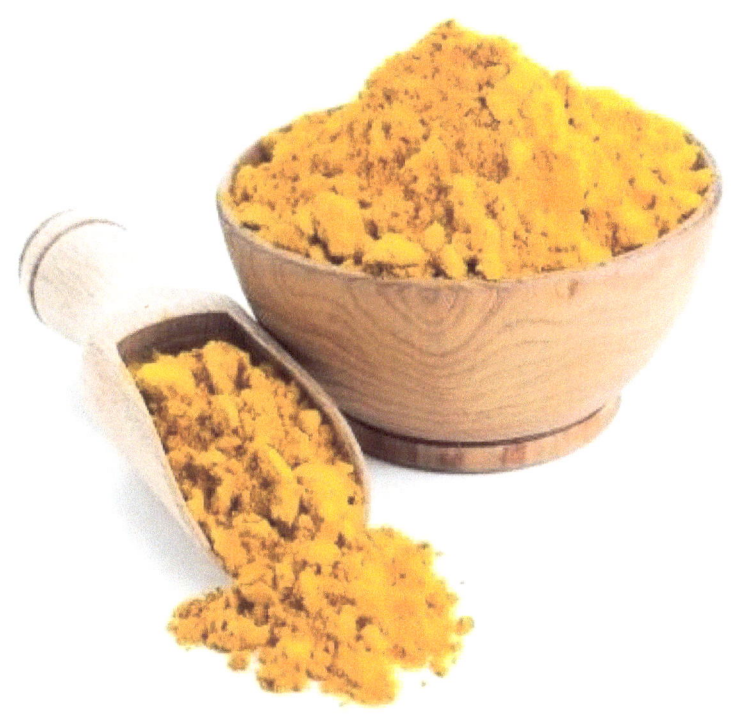

Why is the turmeric roasted? That is because the rhizomes may have some dormant pests invisible to the eye, and yet vulnerable to the heat, which are going to get destroyed by the roasting. This also fixes the color of the turmeric, and once you have ground the powder, all you have to do is place it in an airtight glass jar, and store it in a cool dry place.

This turmeric powder is going to give for anywhere between 6 to 8 weeks, if you continue to give the turmeric a regular airing, in the sun every 15 days or so.

The use of turmeric in the Indian subcontinent goes back millenniums, when the ancient sages, found out that this plant had excellent natural healing qualities. That is why it became an integral part of the Indian lifestyle.

Saffron was extremely expensive, even at that time, and rare. Only royalty and very rich people could afford to add saffron to their food. That was to give the food a golden orangeish tint. But with turmeric easily available to even the common people, every food item could get a luxurious looking rich gold tint at a fraction of the cost. So that is why turmeric became such an important part of a large number of households and this tradition continues throughout the day.

Using Turmeric for Dyeing

Now this is something I found very interesting. I knew that dried onion skins were used since ancient times to dye cotton clothes a light pink, but it is only lately that I found out that turmeric has been used for dyeing clothes a rich saffron color since ancient times.

This is how you do it. Adulterated turmeric powder is going to leave a tinge to the water, if you leave it for 15 minutes after you have stirred a teaspoonful in hot water. Pure turmeric is definitely not going to leave any sort of tint to the water, or if there is something there, it is going to be faintly yellow. Because after all turmeric has a yellow coloring ingredient in it.

But the moment you put it in boiling water, and stir it, it gets ready to dye your clothes a light or darker saffron/yellow color. Let the water cool, and then add 1 tablespoon full of alum in it. This is to preserve the color, so that it does not wash away when you put it in the washing machine and stain all your other clothes.

You may want to soak the clothes, for a little while or for a long while, depending on how deep you want that color. After that, take the cloth out and wash it under a Cold water tap, so that all traces of Alum and turmeric are removed. These clothes are then dried in the shade in the sunny outdoors so that the sun can fix the colors permanently.

So there you are, you can now wear your golden T-shirt, which was white only yesterday.

The only problem with turmeric is that it has this bad habit of staining your clothes, when you use it. Possibly that is the reason why it has not gained popularity in Western kitchens, because the stains are unsightly. Also, when you try to remove them with soap, they turn orange instead of yellow. So I would suggest just rub those stains with lemon juice and salt, and put out in the sun. This is going to bleach the color naturally and get rid of the turmeric.

Stain marks on your T-shirts are definitely going to be a part and parcel of your lifestyle, if you add turmeric to your spice box. So get rid of them naturally. You may need to apply lemon juice and salt, two or three times to get rid of the stain completely.

Turmeric as an Insecticide

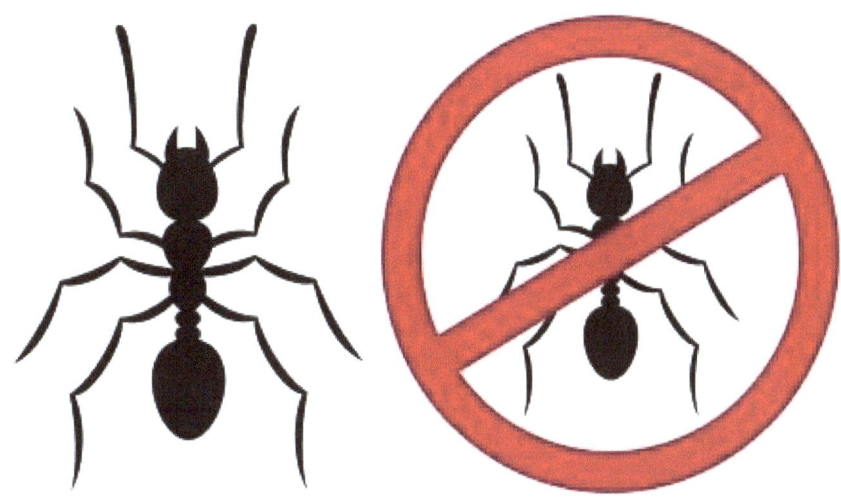

Now just imagine that you have been attacked by an infestation of fans, and other household pests and their making your life miserable. You have ants in your kitchen, you have moths in your cupboard. Do not go in for expensive pesticide remedies when you have easy access to turmeric. Just make a paste of a little bit of turmeric with water, and apply this paste all over the nooks and crannies of the walls.

Turmeric powder, and paste is also considered to be a good natural termite preventative. That is why land on which construction work is going to be done is normally irrigated in the East with a mixture of 1 kg freshly powdered turmeric in a gallon of water. Then the soil is allowed to absorb this amazingly powerful pesticide and get rid of possible termites and ants.

You may want to try this out, especially in doors and windows, which are subject to termite attacks. Just make a paste of turmeric and water, which is going to protect your house from termite in wood and mortar.

The problem with turmeric is that it leaves a stain behind it, especially when you have been using it over a long period of time. So if you have your hands stained with turmeric, just make sure that you are wearing gloves when next you handle it.

Turmeric stains can be removed from your skin by gently rubbing it with warm water and salt.

Apart from that, there are plenty of other uses of turmeric, especially when you want to tint milk products. In fact in the Indian subcontinent, a little bit of turmeric as well as a little bit of salt is added to cottage cheese to preserve it as well as increase its shelf life.

Turmeric for Beauty

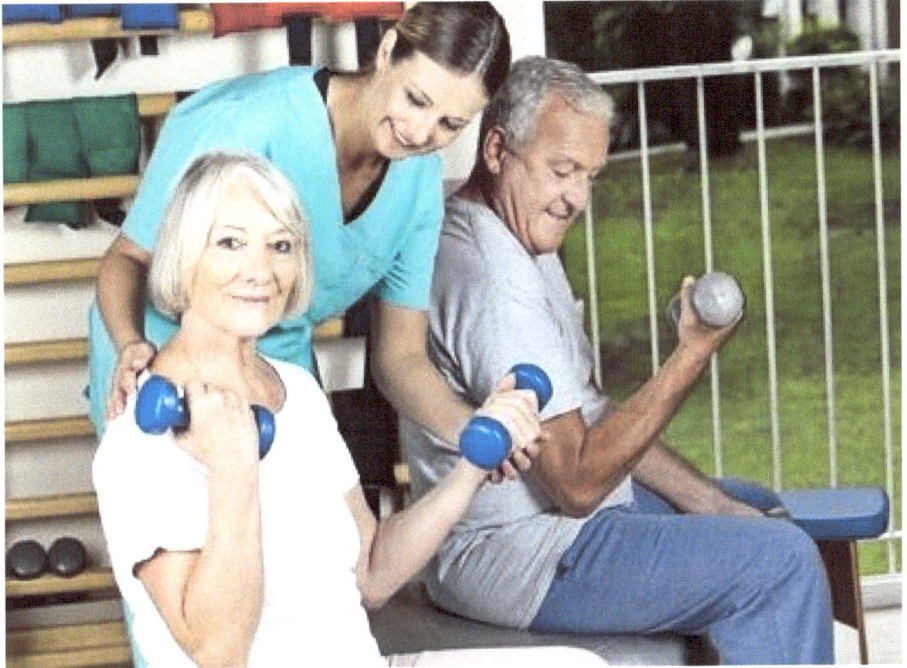

Health conscious? Try turmeric!

Believe it or not, any beautician who is interested in beauty products and natural ingredients which add to your beauty quotient is definitely going to suggest addition of a little bit of turmeric, along with wheat bran, honey, or yogurt and Fullers Earth to any other mixture, in order to make a facemask.

So turmeric stains; but it is also the best antiseptic agent for your skin.

Natural Skin Remedy

Now this young lady cannot stop fiddling with her skin because she thinks that she is suffering from either a possible pimple, a potential wrinkle, or perhaps a blemish. If she applies a paste of turmeric, along with a little bit of milk cream to her skin, as a facemask, and removes it after it has dried, she is going to have a much healthier and much better moisturized skin.

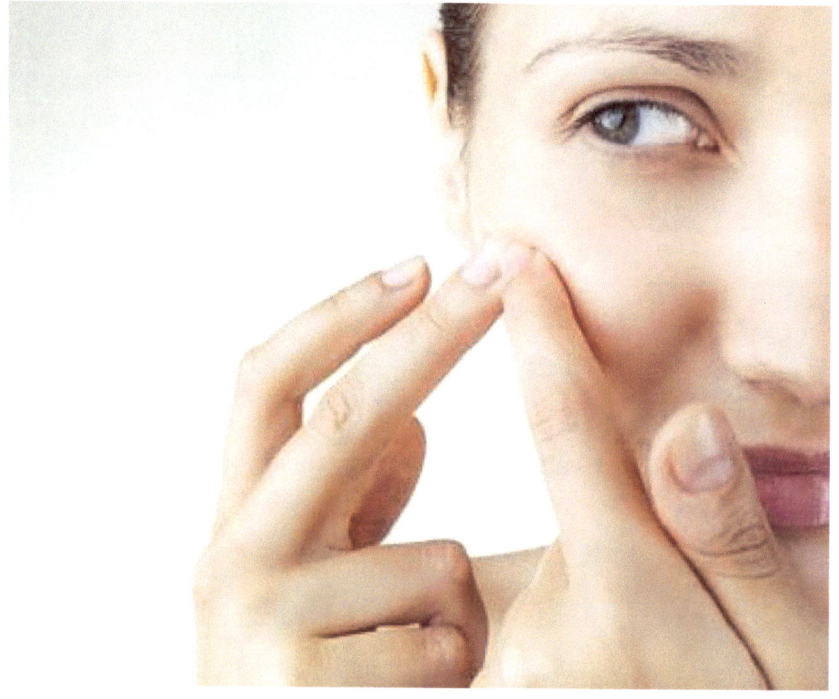

Also, because she is irritating the possible pimple, and making sure that the infection spreads all over her face, she is soon going to suffer from scars. And then she will have to apply turmeric and water paste, all over the scars, in order to lessen their visibility and intensity.

Getting Rid of Skin Blemishes

Now this is a natural facemask, which is used as a cleanser, and moisturizer for your skin, and which will stop you using chemical-based soaps and cleansers. Just add a little bit of turmeric powder to coconut oil, and hot milk – 1 teaspoon each. Now use that as a soap to get rid of all the dust and grime and dead cells. This also clears your complexion, and gets rid of layers of grime, which may cause potential pimples and other skin ailments.

Getting Rid of Sunburn

Sunscreen? Try wearing a hat and then use my sun burn remedy.

Now I am a sun worshiper. I just love soaking in the sun. But the sad side effect of all this spoiling myself is, that I find myself badly sunburned, and also face potential skin damage, which is going to cause me wrinkles when I reach my 60s.

Just add a little bit of turmeric to fresh yogurt, and apply it all over the sunburned area. This is going to bring your skin back to normal. Of course it is going to take a while, but persevere, every day. And keep out of the sun.

Turmeric Body Mask

In the Indian subcontinent, brides have to face a complete body mask, made up of turmeric, chickpea powder, coconut, or almond oil, and sandalwood powder. This is done for one week before the wedding ceremony every evening when all the bride's friends gather around her.

Of course, the sandalwood is extremely expensive, but you can get the same effect by leaving out the sandalwood, and using the rest of the ingredients to scrub your skin from top to toe.

Oatmeal Turmeric Scrub

Try using an oatmeal scrub with a little bit of turmeric and a little bit of milk cream on that rough skin on your elbows, neck and knees. This is going to smoothen it out, and it is also going to refresh you. Apply this 20 minutes before you take your shower, and by the time, the hot water is ready for your shower, the oatmeal and turmeric will have dried. You are now slowly going to rub it off to get healthy, glistening, smooth and well moisturized skin.

Turmeric in a Toothpaste?

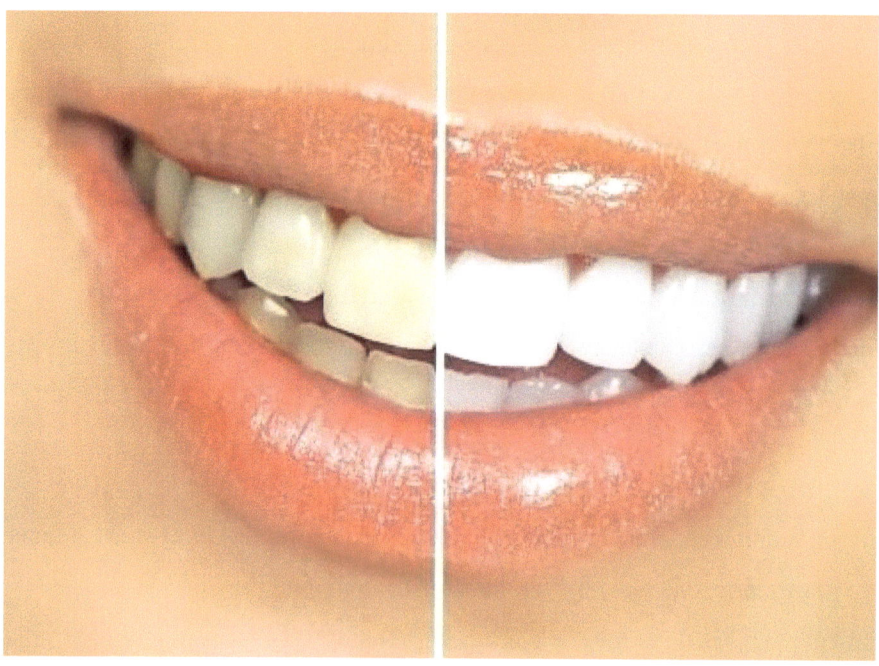

Believe it or not, turmeric, along with salt and a touch of asafetida has been in use to keep teeth healthy, and you should be astonished to know that former beauty queen Susie Castillo has revealed that she used her own homemade toothpaste that contained turmeric to whiten her teeth.

This may come as a surprise to many people due to the color of turmeric but turmeric does work as a teeth whitener. But you need to make sure that it does not remain in contact with the teeth for over 30 minutes.

So what is your turmeric toothpaste going to be made of? So here I am, giving up beauty secrets used by beauty queens, but which have managed to keep her teeth shining white like those of her ancestors.

This toothpaste is going to consist of a mixture of 1 teaspoon each of salt, soda bicarbonate, and lemon juice along with four large pinches of turmeric powder. You can either dip your toothbrush in this mixture, and rub it all over your teeth, to bleach them or you can do something really messier. You can add mustard oil, and half a teaspoonful of black pepper as well as some clove oil, to prevent any sort of tooth infection in the future.

So it really does not matter whether you are using your toothpaste to bleach your teeth or for preventing any sort of mouth and gum infection; turmeric is going to be a part of that procedure. Brush your teeth for not more than one minute twice every day with this natural toothpaste/gum massage mixture.

Remember to roast the turmeric before you powder it.

Once that is done, and you have been using this toothpaste, you can enjoy many enjoyable turmeric and health-based dishes like those given on the following pages.

Sprouted Lentil Veggie Burger

Ingredients:

2 cups sprouted lentils

1 cooked, mashed sweet potato

2 tablespoons butter

3 tablespoons ground flax

1 teaspoon turmeric

2 cloves

1 teaspoon salt

1 teaspoon pepper

Directions:

Before starting to make this burger, make sure you have sprouted red lentils.

Cook the sweet potatoes in a 400 degrees oven, remove their skin and mash them.

Combine the ingredients in a food processor and mix them.

Form the mix into patties and cook them in a skillet using butter or oil. After the one half has browned, flip and cook the other half.

Serve with avocado, cheese or any other of your favorite toppings.

Orange Turmeric Cake

Ingredients:

250 grams butter

250 grams sugar

4 eggs

150 grams Greek yogurt

20 grams turmeric powder

200 grams almond meal

150 grams polenta

1 teaspoon baking (bicarb) soda

2 oranges

½ cup of thick Greek yogurt

½ cup icing sugar

Orange zest to garnish

Directions:

Pre-heat your oven to 180 degrees Celsius.

Line a 20cm, circular baking tin with baking paper, apply butter to it and coat it with polenta. In a mixing bowl, cream the sugar and butter till it turns pale. Add one egg at a time and mix it till it combines; add and stir the turmeric and yogurt.

Add the almond meal, baking (bicarb) soda and polenta and mix them. Then add the zest and juice from the oranges and stir them together.

Bake in an oven for 1 hour. After five minutes of cooling turn out the cake. Allow the cake to cool for an hour before icing it.

Combine the icing sugar & yogurt and spread it over the top of the cake.

Marinated Grilled Prawns

Now this is something which is going to be enjoyed by people who really love seafood. I cannot resist it, especially when it is grilled and I do not have to worry about the fat content. This is excellent for snacks, especially when you're serving it with drinks.

When a friend made this traditionally, she did not bother about de-shelling the prawns, and deveining them. She said the crunch quotient made eating these fun. Not for me! I like them shelled before I add them to the marinade.

For all those who want to know how to shell prawns – enjoy

http://www.youtube.com/watch?v=i8dkFz1cuzU

but he did not show you how to devein them.

For that you need to go here –
http://www.youtube.com/watch?v=yyaKOl1ZjLM

I normally use the knife to make a slit on the back and front of the prawns, and then scoop out the veins. Whatever works!

Seriously speaking, I asked a fisherman, whether these were veins, and he said completely blank faced, no, they were the algae eaten by the prawns. Well, they were green enough!

1 kg of uncooked king prawns
One medium onion chopped
Half a cup of plain yogurt
Half a teaspoonful of ground turmeric
Half a teaspoon of chili powder
1 tablespoon of paprika
1 teaspoon grated fresh ginger
Two cloves of garlic crushed
1 tablespoon full of lemon juice

Wash the prawns which you may or may not have shelled and deveined and pat them dry with absorbent paper. Blend and process the yogurt, turmeric, onion, paprika, chili powder, garlic, ginger and the lemon juice until it is smooth.

Combine the prawns and the spicy yogurt mixture in a bowl, cover after you have mixed well, and allowed to refrigerate overnight. This means that the marinade is going to have plenty of time to work its magic.

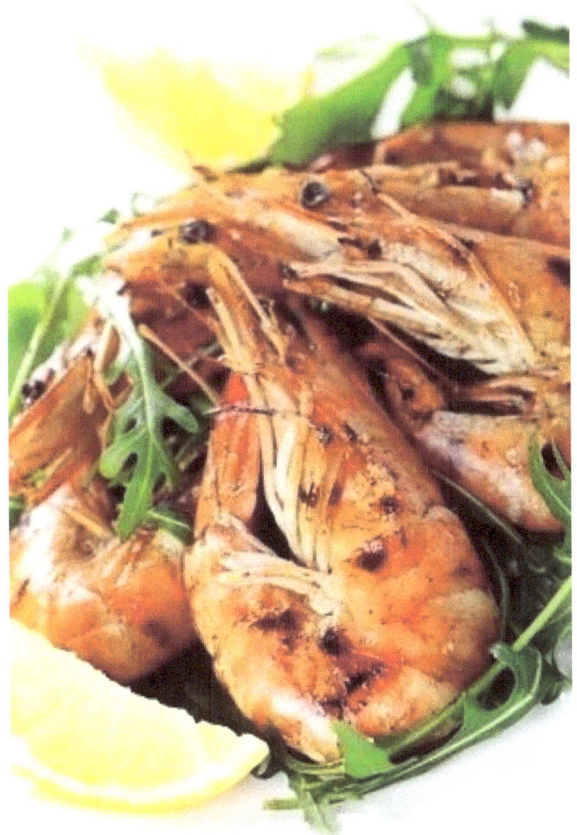

Remove the bowl on the day of grilling, or barbecuing, and allowed to come to room temperature before you put them on the grill. Grill till they are tender. You may want to brush occasionally with the marinade when they are cooking.

Serve with onion rings and capsicum.

Savory Chickpeas

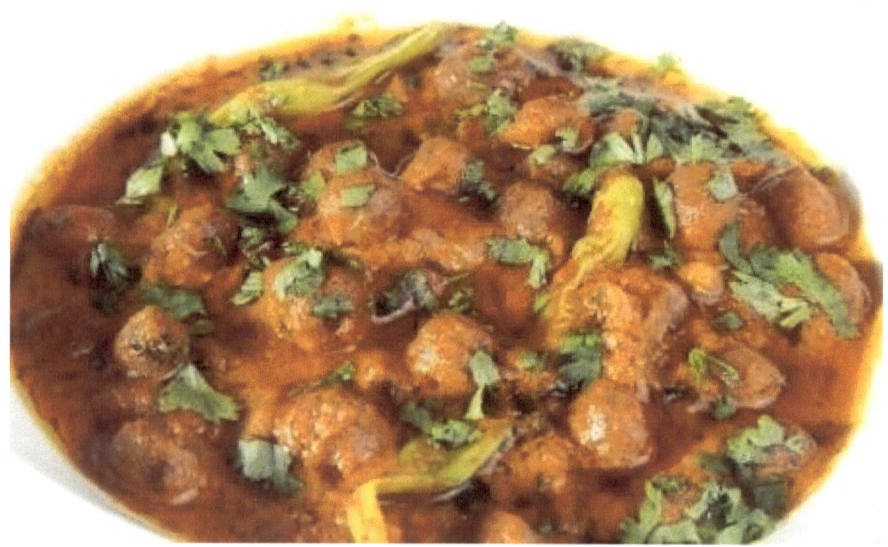

Now this is an extremely healthy dish, which is going to add more variety to your meals. It is eaten extensively all over the Indian subcontinent, with roti, and at every party, the guest is going to feel cheated, if he doesn't find any meat dish in curry form, basmati rice and chickpeas for the vegetarians.

So for this dish you need:

2 cups chickpeas

1 tablespoon full of cumin seeds,

2 tablespoons shredded ginger

One teaspoonful of salt

One large potato, peeled and cubed after boiling

Five – 6 teaspoons of oil for cooking

And one tablespoonful of clarified butter for seasoning.

After that, you need a marinade of half a teaspoonful of garam masala powder

1 teaspoon of coriander powder

1 teaspoon of red chili powder

1 ½ teaspoon dried pomegranate seeds, coarsely ground,

1 teaspoon salt

And garnish with two green chilies, one medium-sized tomato cut into rings, one small onion cut into rings, one lemon cut into wedges.

Watch the chickpeas and place in a bowl to soak overnight with 1 teaspoon salt after you have covered it with water. This is going to lessen the cooking time, which you would normally spend getting those chickpeas to boil to perfection. In many parts of India, they had a little bit of soda bicarbonate to the water before the overnight soaking, but that is overkill.

Drain the chickpeas and rinse in a number of changes of water, so that all the white bubbly impurities is rising up to the top are removed completely.

Place the chickpeas in a pressure cooker, with 1 L of water and cook for 40 to 45 minutes until they are cooked properly. Now for those people who are not accustomed to cooking with pressure cookers, getting these chickpeas to boil properly is a headache. It is going to take one to two hours on full heat and the water boiling over occasionally. Under such circumstances you need to put just enough of water to cover them, and keep watching to see that the chickpeas have not gotten burnt.

Open cooker when it is cool, drain the chickpeas and reserve the cooking liquid.

Combine all the ingredients for the marinade in a bowl. When the chickpeas are cooled, add to the marinade bowl, with ginger, cumin seeds, potato and oil. Mix this well and set aside for three hours.

Now transfer the contents of the bowl to your Wok and place over low heat. Add 1 cup from the reserved chickpea liquid, and simmer over low heat for another 30 minutes.

Remove from the heat, and spoon into your serving bowl. Drizzle hot clarified butter also known as desi ghee right on top and garnish with tomato, onions, chilies and lemon wedges. This is best eaten piping hot with rice or bread.

Turmeric to Heal You

Turmeric has long been known as a natural healer, which is going to get rid of any problems in your tummy, and in your intestines. That is why if you are suffering from any such ailments, you are going to be advised to drink turmeric, mixed up with buttermilk. Just add three large pinches of roasted turmeric to rock salt to taste in your glassful of buttermilk. Drink this as often as possible. Not only is buttermilk going to heal any sort of infection in your stomach, but so will turmeric heal you.

Since ancient times, this buttermilk and turmeric remedy was used to treat people suffering from dysentery and diarrhea. The salt prevented them from getting dehydrated. Also, people suffering from flatulence can use this remedy to get rid of any sort of flatulence related problems, even if it is chronic.

Tummy Parasites?

This is of course an occupational hazard with a lot of children, especially when they are not bothered much about washing the fruit, they eat. That is why they find themselves suffering from tummy parasites which cause them to grind their teeth at night when asleep, and as tradition says, even talk at night, because the parasites are moving around in their digestive system!

Of course, tomato with freshly ground pepper, eaten first thing in the morning for three days is an excellent way in which you can get rid of these parasites. You do not have to go in for deworming tablets. The other ancient cure for getting rid of these parasites is to take one teaspoonful of raw rhizome turmeric juice with a little bit of salt. Take this first thing in the morning just once a day. You will need to repeat this, three times, and on the third morning, you are going to see those parasites being eliminated from your system.

Suffering from anemia?

Now this is a question I want to ask researchers, who are researching on the magic of turmeric, but have not bothered to find out about its qualities, to cure potential anemia and possible blood related diseases. Just take turmeric juice, 1 teaspoon, with one teaspoonful of honey once every day until you find yourself getting better and your red blood corpuscles increasing in their count.

Turmeric for Curing Wounds

Now this is an ancient remedy, which is known by wise women down the millenniums, especially when their men folk were warriors. So when they came staggering back after slight skirmishes with the neighborhood warriors, bringing back loot and possibly infected wounds, the women went into action mode.

All the wounds, whether they were infected or not, were first cleaned with boiling water to make sure that there was no dirt remaining. Since ancient times in the East, it has been known that wounds have to be washed out with water in which a little bit of salt is added, and never mind the screaming.

When the soldiers did not have turmeric on their battlegrounds, they just picked up some ash from their cooking ovens, and spread it all over the wound in order to prevent infection. And when they came home, the women cleaned the wounds, and bandaged them again, after they put on a paste of turmeric, with water and bandaging with a clean cotton cloth.

Believe it or not, I use this method to cure myself, when I suffer from sprains, torn muscles, and any internal injuries. I just stagger back home, get a glassful of milk from the refrigerator, put it on to boil and add a teaspoonful of raw turmeric powder to it when still boiling. Then I drink it down red-hot, with a teaspoonful of honey added.

I don't know whether this is autosuggestion, or whether turmeric really works to cure my torn tissues, but this is in use for centuries, and the milk and the turmeric is considered to be super efficacious in every such case.

This also prevents your body from swelling up due to shock, and of course, the muscular tissues are going to enjoy that nice drink of milk. I just drink one glass every day, because I don't take more than one – two teaspoonful of turmeric, throughout a day.

Turmeric Antiseptic

If you are in the Indian subcontinent, and you do not have access to a doctor, and you are moving about in rural areas, and you manage to get yourself hurt, the nearest villager is going to say it is nothing – just apply some turmeric paste.

So I'm giving you an excellent turmeric paste, which you can make, and put in a small glass box, and take all over the corner of the compass, reassured of the fact that you are never going to suffer from any sort of infections through wounds, cuts and bruises.

Just take hundred grams of coconut oil. Allow to boil. Add one teaspoonful of roasted powdered turmeric to this oil. Now takes 10 g of beeswax and melt over hot water. Now add the turmeric oil to this antiseptic coconut until you have an ointment. Allow to cool, and then pour in your glass bottle.

The next time you suffer from any sort of injury, just scoop up a finger full of this ointment, and apply over the cleaned area. Then slap on a bandage and forget about it, till tomorrow, when you're going to repeat this process again until you are completely cured.

Remember injuries get very easily infected in tropical regions. So never neglect any sort of injury, when you are climbing up mountains and down dales, saying that your doctor is going to take care of that, when you reach civilization in about a week or so. By then, many times the wound gets badly infected and even gangrenous.

Turmeric and Onions team up against Colon Cancer

A research published in the 2006 issue of Clinical Gastroenterology and Hematology concluded that curcumin found in turmeric and quercitin, an anti-oxidant compound in onions can reduce the size as well as number of precancerous abnormalities in the intestinal tracts of humans.

Five patients with an inherited case of precancerous tissue abnormalities in the lower bowel region were given regular doses of quercitin and curcumin over a period of six months. After six months the numbers of tissue abnormalities dropped by 60.4% while their size dropped by 50.9%.

These abnormalities found in the lower bowel are known as familial adenomatous polyposis or FAP. As the name suggests, FAP runs in families and involves the development of hundreds of tissues that eventually become fully cancerous cells.

Lead researcher Francis M. Giariello at the Gastroenterology division at John Hopkins states that in recent times anti-inflammatory drugs such as ibuprofen and aspirin have been used to treat these conditions but the idea is being discouraged due to their serious side effects that include gastrointestinal bleedings and ulcerations.

Observational studies at a macro level have shown that societies that consume large amounts of turmeric rich foods have lower cases of intestinal problems such as colon cancer. Similarly, quercitin that is present mainly in onions and green tea has been found to subdue the growth of cancerous cells in humans.

Conclusion

Everything you need to know about turmeric has been given in this book, from its history to its recipes, its medicinal worth and household use. This spice has innumerable benefits and if one can incorporate it in his/her daily routine, it can do wonders.

Since it has no serious, life-threatening side-effect it can be consumed with no worries. In fact, it can make a lot of foods more appetizing and delicious.

So keep turmeric close to yourself and lead a healthy life.

Live long and prosper!

Author Bio

Dueep Jyot Singh is a Management and IT Professional who managed to gather Postgraduate qualifications in Management and English and Degrees in Science, French and Education while pursuing different enjoyable career options like being an hospital administrator, IT,SEO and HRD Database Manager/ trainer, movie scriptwriter, theatre artiste and public speaker, lecturer in French, Marketing and Advertising, ex-Editor of Hearts On Fire (now known as Solstice) Books Missouri USA, advice columnist and cartoonist, publisher and Aviation School trainer, ex- moderator on Medico.in, banker, student councilor ,travelogue writer … among other things! One fine morning, she decided that she had enough of killing herself by Degrees and went back to her first love -- writing. It's more enjoyable! She already has 48 published academic and 14 fiction- in- different- genre books under her belt.

When she is not designing websites or making Graphic design illustrations for clients , she is browsing through old bookshops hunting for treasures, of which she has an enviable collection – including R.L. Stevenson, O.Henry, Dornford Yates, Maurice Walsh, C.N.Williamson, Sapper, Bartimeus and the crown of her collection- Dickens "The Old Curiosity Shop," and so on… Just call her "Renaissance Woman" - collecting herbal remedies, acting like Universal Helping Hand/Agony Aunt, or escaping to her dear mountains for a bit of exploring, collecting herbs and plants, and trekking.

Check out some of the other JD-Biz Publishing books
Health Learning Series

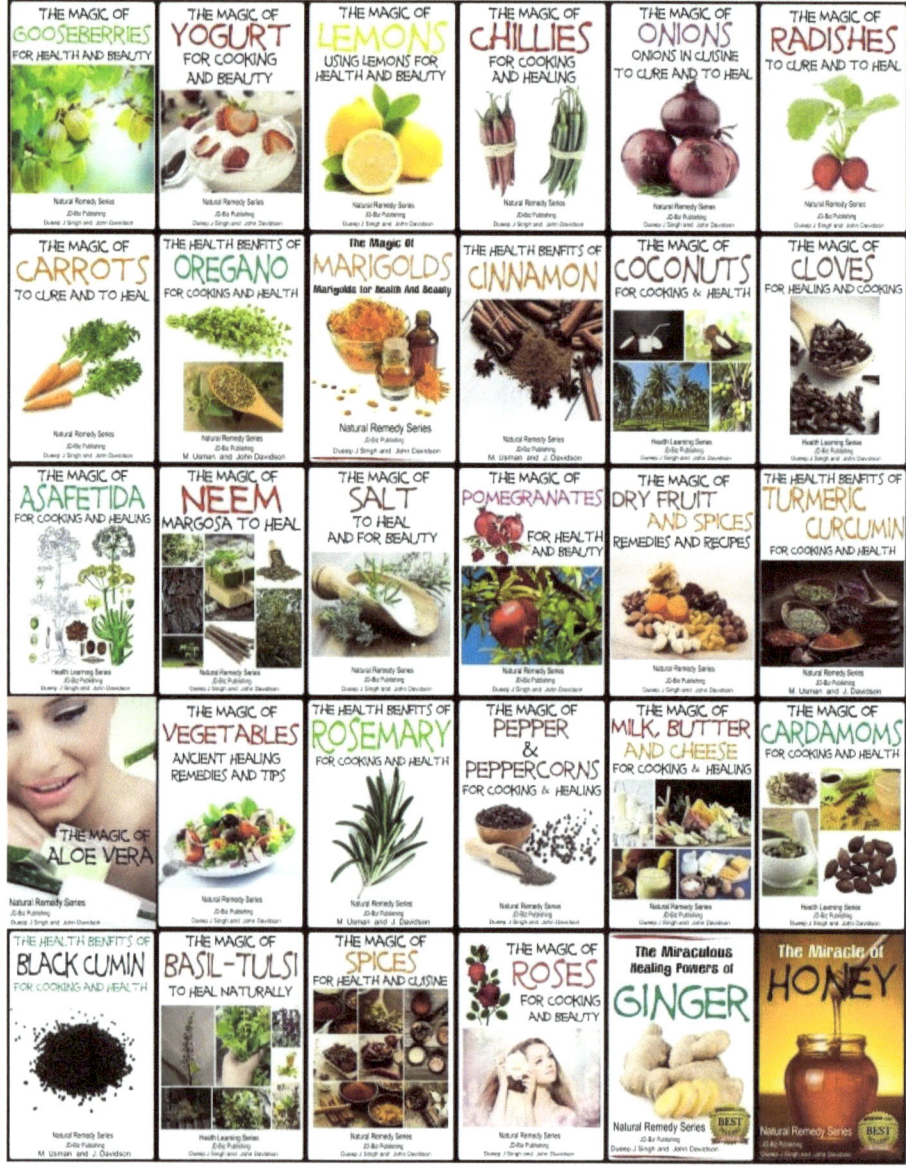

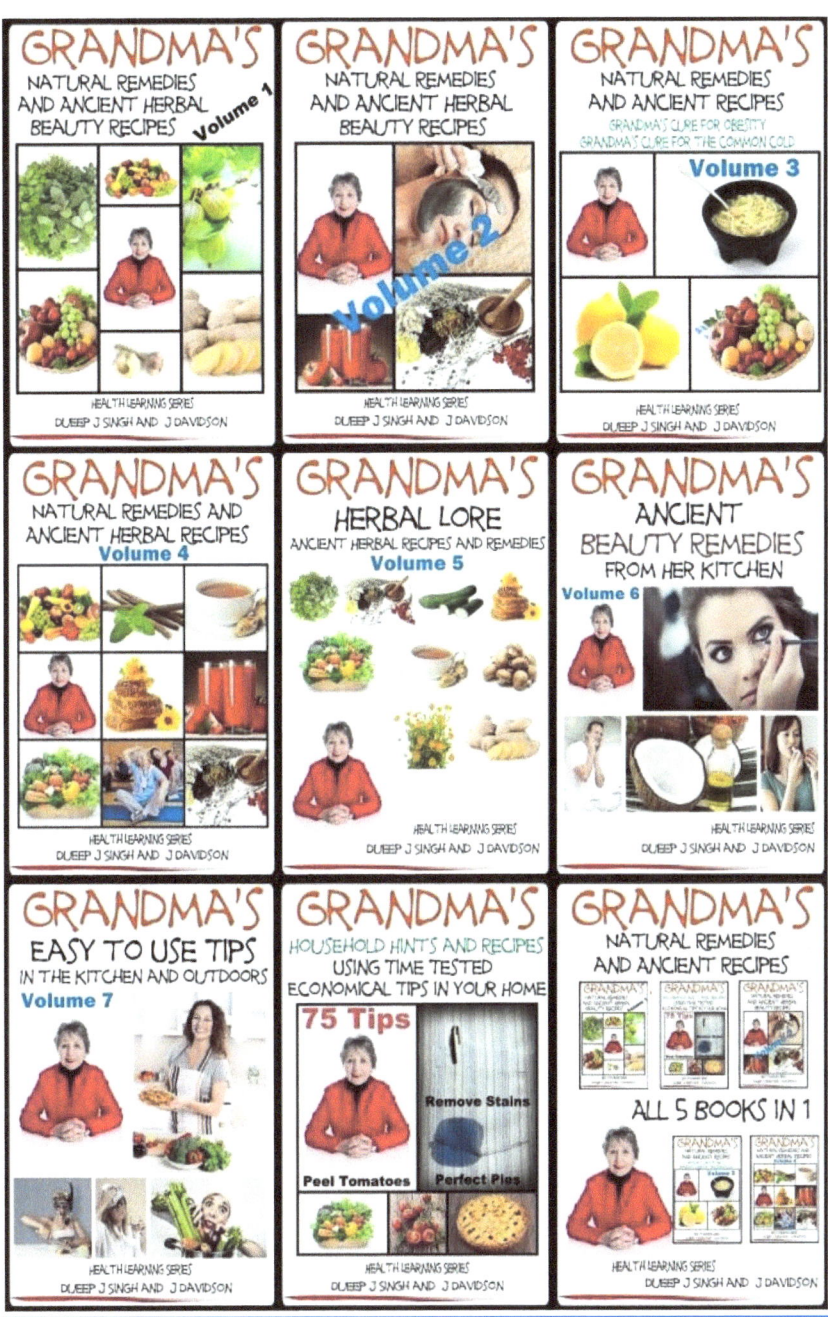

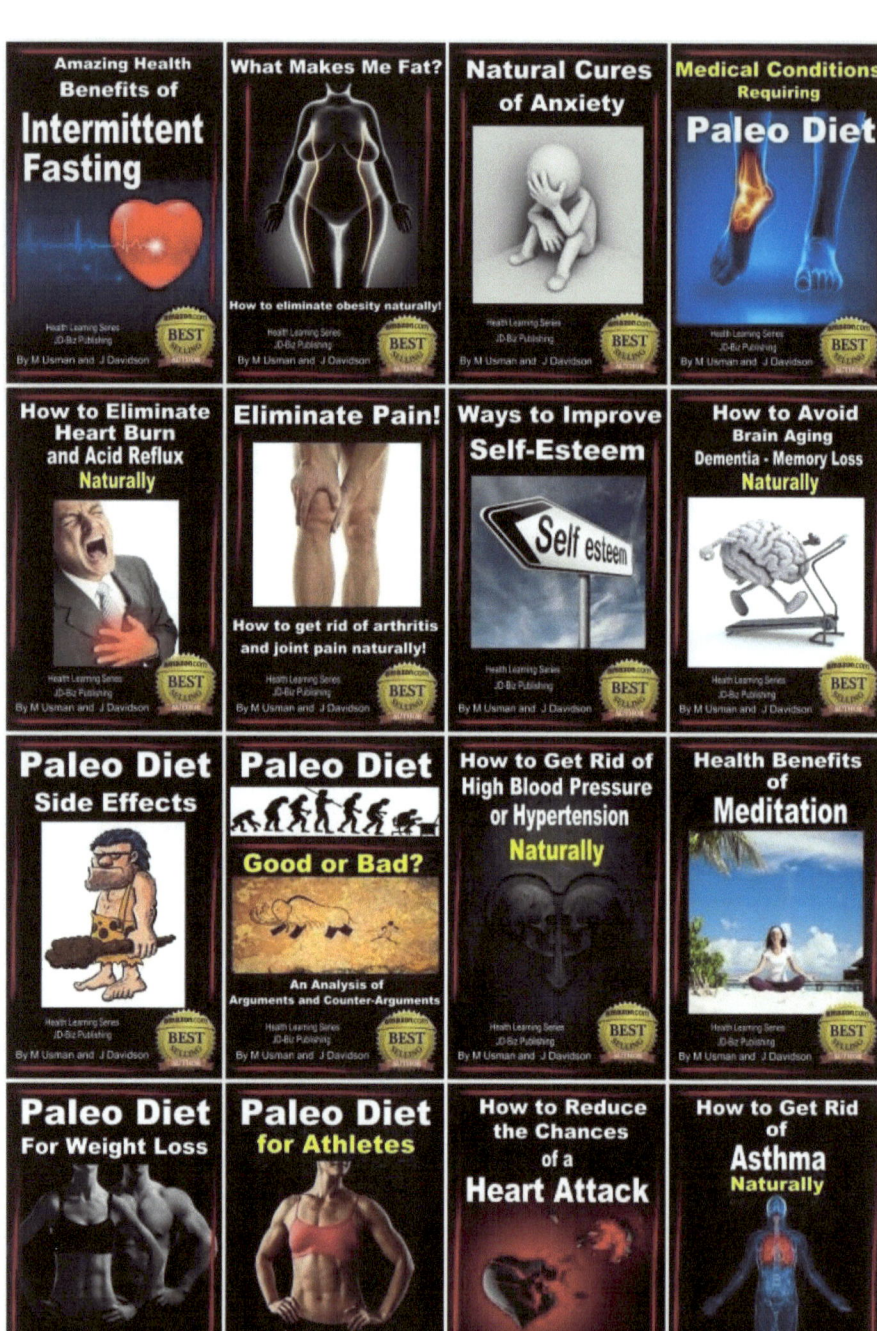

Amazing Animal Book Series

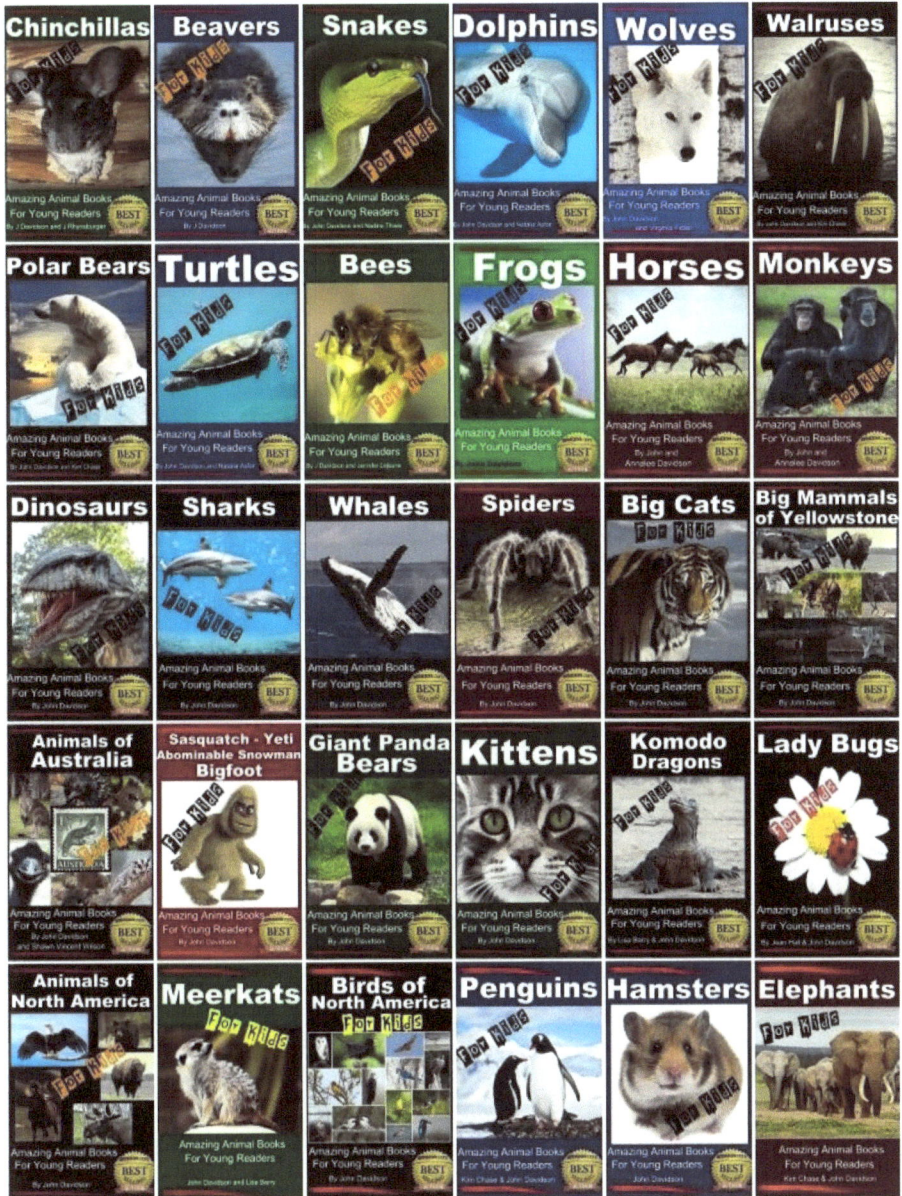

Learn To Draw Series

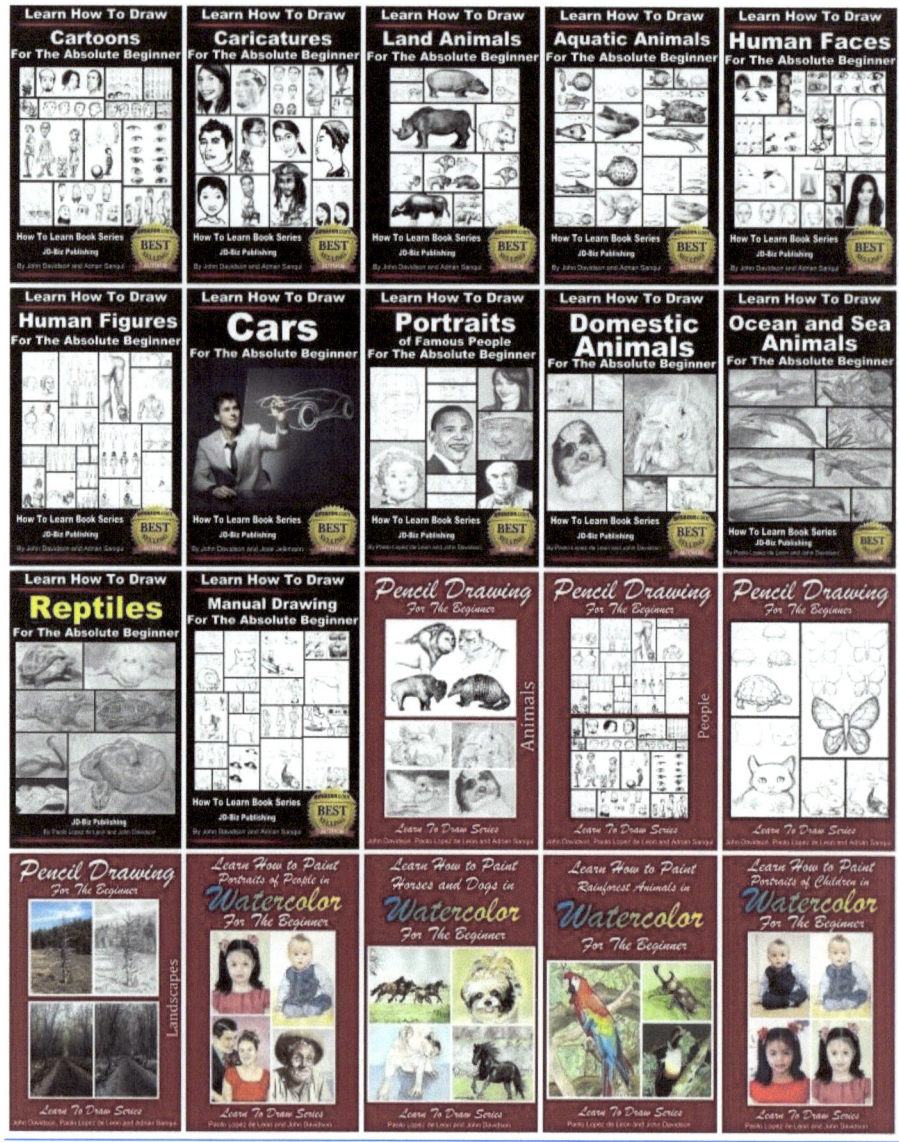

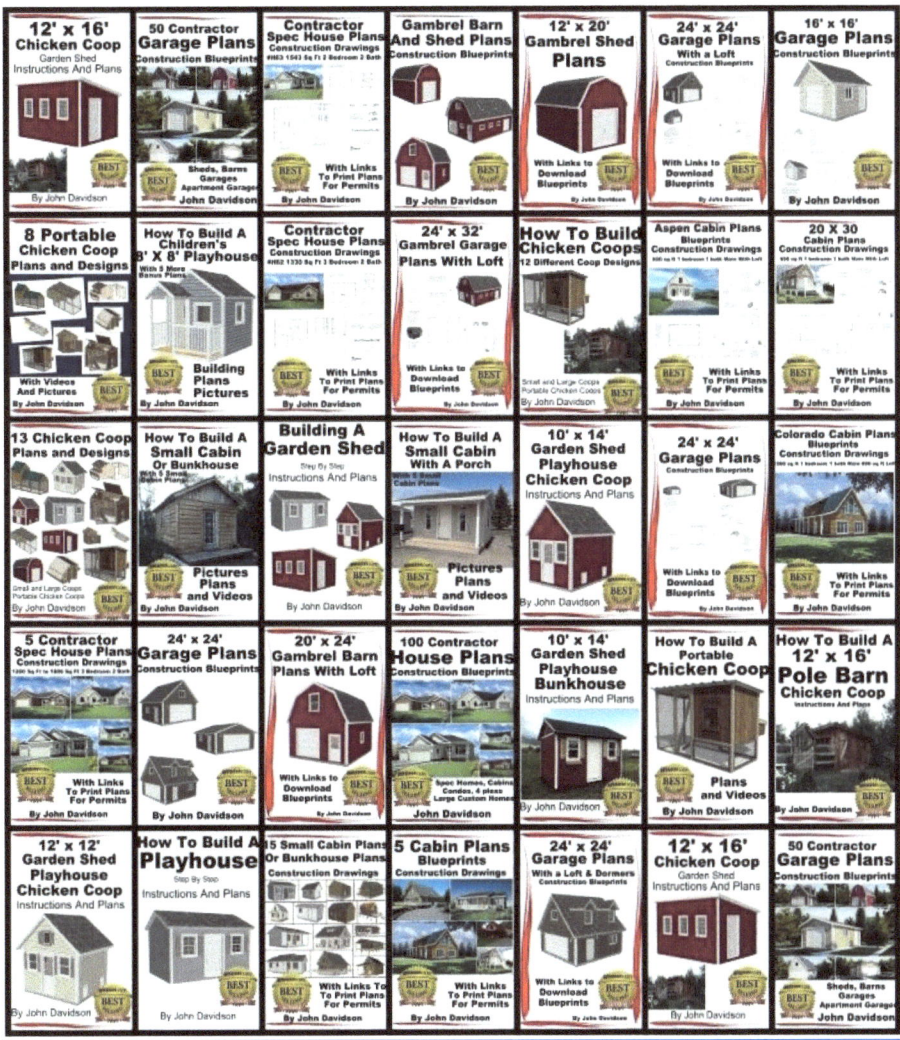

Entrepreneur Book Series

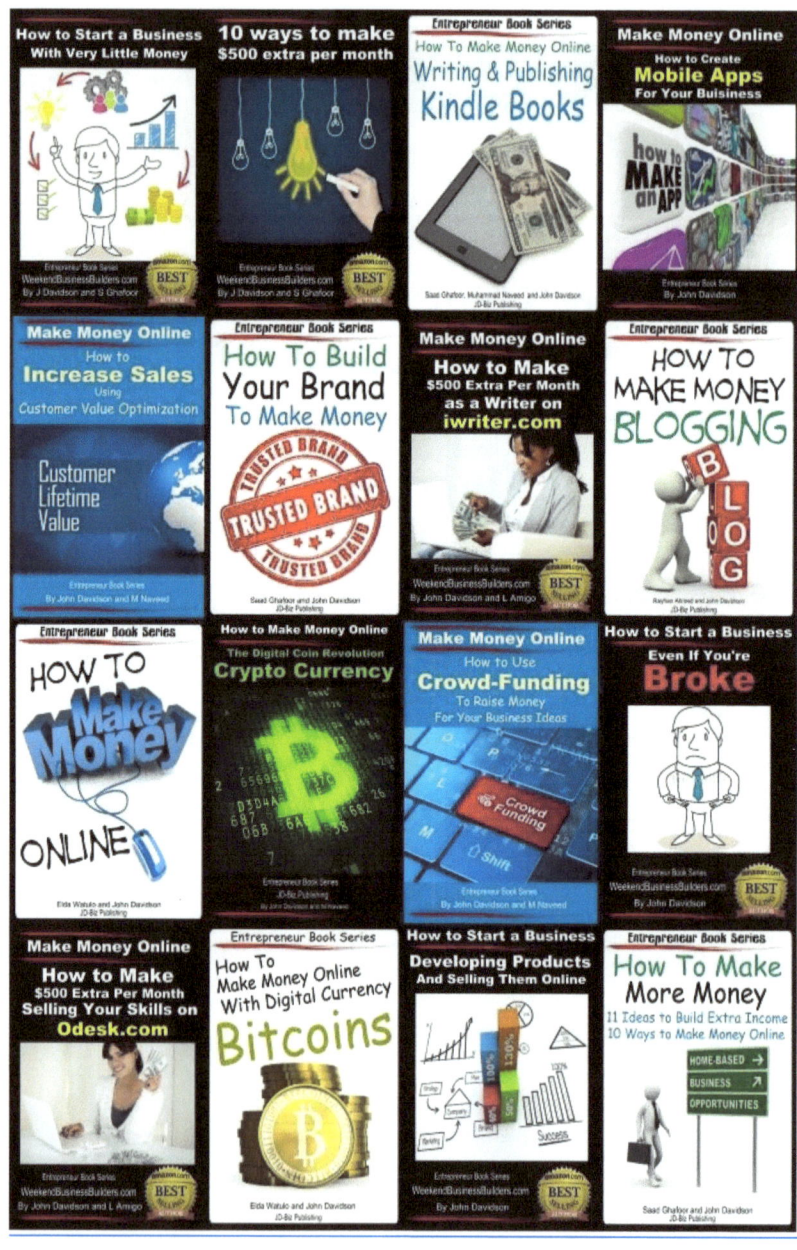

Our books are available at

1. Amazon.com

2. Barnes and Noble

3. Itunes

4. Kobo

5. Smashwords

6. Google Play Books

Download Free Books!

http://MendonCottageBooks.com

Publisher

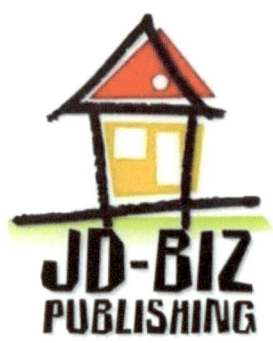

JD-Biz Corp

P O Box 374

Mendon, Utah 84325

http://www.jd-biz.com/

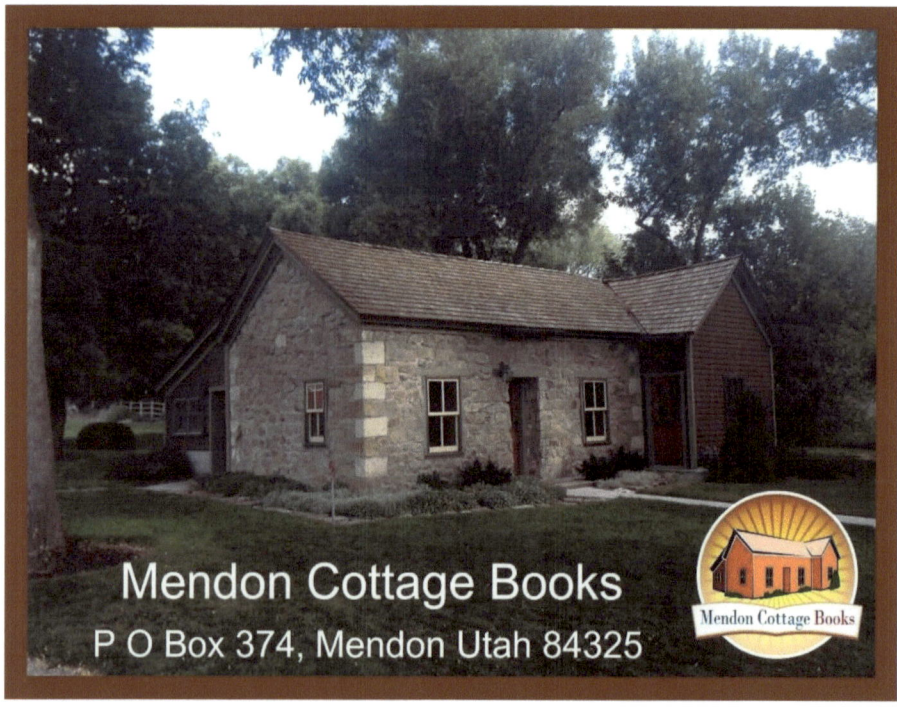

Mendon Cottage Books

P O Box 374, Mendon Utah 84325

www.ingramcontent.com/pod-product-compliance
Lightning Source LLC
Chambersburg PA
CBHW050836290526
45792CB00001B/418